67 Organic Kidney Disease Juice Recipes:

Solve Your Kidney Problems without Pills or Medicine

By

Joe Correa CSN

COPYRIGHT

ACKNOWLEDGEMENTS

This book is dedicated to my friends and family that have had mild or serious illnesses so that you may find a solution and make the necessary changes in your life.

67 Organic Kidney Disease Juice Recipes:

Solve Your Kidney Problems without Pills or Medicine

By

Joe Correa CSN

CONTENTS

ABOUT THE AUTHOR

After years of Research, I honestly believe in the positive effects that proper nutrition can have over the body and mind. My knowledge and experience has helped me live healthier throughout the years and which I have shared with family and friends. The more you know about eating and drinking healthier, the sooner you will want to change your life and eating habits.

Nutrition is a key part in the process of being healthy and living longer so get started today. The first step is the most important and the most significant.

INTRODUCTION

67 Organic Kidney Disease Juice Recipes: Solve Your Kidney Problems without Pills or Medicine

By Joe Correa CSN

As you probably already know, healthy kidneys help remove different kinds of waste and fluids from the body through urine. This waste usually includes chemicals, medication, and other substances that remain in the blood after digestion. Furthermore, healthy kidneys produce an active form of vitamin D, regulate the balance of water and different minerals like phosphorus, potassium, and sodium in the blood, and produce a chemical substance called renin. Renin is used by the body to regulate blood pressure.

Kidney disease is defined as any form of abnormality in these organs. These abnormalities prevent normal kidney function and lead to some serious medical conditions, mainly waste products are kept inside your body. Without a proper treatment, kidney disease can lead to complete kidney failure and a life-threatening condition.

The main causes of kidney disease are diabetes, high blood pressure, urinary tract infections, overuse of different drugs, inherited kidney disease, and of course an unhealthy diet based on highly processed foods full of different chemicals. In order to keep your kidneys healthy and prevent complications, you need to learn how to recognize the first symptoms related to kidney disease. These symptoms include poor sleep, swelling in your ankles, vomiting, overall weakness and lack of energy, shortness of breath, and urination problems. All of these symptoms should be examined by your physician to determine their cause.

Just like every other medical condition, kidney disease is closely related to a poor diet and an unhealthy lifestyle. Researchers have discovered numerous links between inflammation and some foods that are able to prevent chronic and degenerative conditions. Foods like bell peppers, cabbage, cauliflower, garlic, apples, cranberries, blueberries, raspberries, cherries, and grapes are rich in antioxidants that are able to neutralize free radicals and protect the body. These foods are the basis of a healthy, kidney-friendly diet and should be included in your meals and juices every day.

For this reason, I have created these delicious juice recipes based on ingredients that are proven to clean the body and improve kidney function. These recipes are designed to easily fit in your daily schedule and satisfy even the most demanding taste buds. Have your dose of nutrients every single day and give your kidneys what they need to function properly!

67 ORGANIC KIDNEY DISEASE JUICE RECIPES: SOLVE YOUR KIDNEY PROBLEMS WITHOUT PILLS OR MEDICINE

1.   Apple Lemon Juice

Ingredients:

1 small Golden Delicious apple, cored and chopped

1 whole lemon, peeled and halved

1 cup of pumpkin, cubed

1 large carrot, sliced

1 cup of watercress, torn

Preparation:

Wash the apple and cut lengthwise in half. Remove the core and cut into bite-sized pieces. Set aside.

Peel the lemon and cut lengthwise in half. Set aside.

Cut the top of a pumpkin. Cut lengthwise in half and then scrape out the seeds. Cut one large wedge and peel it. Cut into small cubes and fill the measuring cup. Reserve the rest in the refrigerator.

Wash and peel the carrot. Cut into thin slices and set aside.

Rinse the watercress thoroughly under cold running water. Drain and torn into small pieces. Set aside.

Now, combine apple, lemon, pumpkin, carrot, and watercress in a juicer and process until juiced. Transfer to a serving glass and add some ice before serving.

Enjoy!

Nutrition information per serving: Kcal: 126, Protein: 3.6g, Carbs: 37.8g, Fats: 0.7g

2.   Pineapple Spinach Juice

Ingredients:

1 cup of pineapple, chunked

1 cup of spinach, chopped

1 cup of cherries, pitted

1 whole lemon, peeled

¼ tsp of cinnamon, ground

1 oz of water

Preparation:

Using a sharp paring knife, cut the top of the pineapple. Gently remove all hard skin and slice it into thin slices. Fill the measuring cup and reserve the rest for later.

Rinse the spinach thoroughly under cold running water. Drain and chop into small pieces. Set aside.

Place the cherries in a medium colander. Rinse well under cold running water and remove the stems, if any. Cut each in half and remove the pits. Fill the measuring cup and reserve the rest in the refrigerator.

Peel the lemon and cut lengthwise in half. Set aside.

Now, combine pineapple, spinach, cherries, and lemon in a juicer and process until juiced. Transfer to a serving glass and stir in the water.

Add some crushed ice and serve immediately.

Nutrition information per serving: Kcal: 196, Protein: 9.2g, Carbs: 59.3g, Fats: 1.5g

3.   Cantaloupe Cucumber Juice

Ingredients:

1 cup of cantaloupe, peeled and chopped

1 large cucumber

1 cup of avocado, peeled and pitted

1 large lemon, peeled

Preparation:

Cut the cantaloupe in half. Scoop out the seeds and flesh. Cut two wedges and peel them. Chop into chunks and set aside. Reserve the rest of the cantaloupe in a refrigerator.

Wash the cucumber and cut into thick slices. Set aside.

Peel the avocado and cut in half. Remove the pit and cut into chunks. Set aside.

Peel the lemon and cut in half. Set aside.

Now, process cantaloupe, cucumber, avocado, and lemon in a juicer.

Transfer to serving glasses and add some water to adjust the thickness, if needed.

Add some ice and serve immediately.

Nutritional information per serving: Kcal: 292, Protein: 6.8g, Carbs: 41.5g, Fats: 22.2g

4.   Parsnip Carrot Juice

Ingredients:

1 cup of parsnip, sliced

1 large carrot, sliced

1 cup of cauliflower, chopped

1 cup of fennel, trimmed and chopped

1 whole lime, peeled

Preparation:

Wash and peel the parsnip and carrot. Cut into thin slices and fill the measuring cup. Reserve the rest for later.

Wash the cauliflower and trim off the outer leaves. Cut into small pieces and fill the measuring cup. Reserve the rest for later.

Trim off the fennel stalks and outer wilted layers. Wash and chop the fennel into bite-sized pieces. Fill the measuring cup and reserve the rest for later. Set aside.

Peel the lime and cut lengthwise in half. Set aside.

Now, combine parsnip, carrot, cauliflower, fennel, and lime in a juicer. Process until well juiced.

Transfer to a serving glass and refrigerate for 10 minutes before serving.

Add some turmeric or ginger for some extra taste. However, it's optional.

Nutrition information per serving: Kcal: 141, Protein: 5.6g, Carbs: 46.2g, Fats: 1.1g

5. Grapefruit Broccoli Juice

Ingredients:

1 large grapefruit, peeled

1 cup of broccoli

1 large apricot, pitted

1 large banana

Preparation:

Peel the grapefruit and cut into bite-sized pieces. Set aside.

Place the broccoli in a colander and wash under cold running water. Chop into small pieces and set aside.

Wash the apricot and cut in half. Remove the pit and cut into small pieces. Set aside.

Peel the banana and cut into small chunks. Set aside.

Now, process grapefruit, broccoli, apricot, and banana in a juicer. Transfer to serving glasses and refrigerate for 30 minutes before serving.

Nutritional information per serving: Kcal: 229, Protein: 6.5g, Carbs: 67.2g, Fats: 1.3g

6. Brussels Sprout Parsley Juice

Ingredients:

1 cup of Brussels sprouts, chopped

1 cup of parsley, chopped

2 whole leeks, chopped

2 whole kiwis, chopped

A handful of spinach, chopped

½ cup of water

Preparation:

Wash the Brussels sprouts and trim off the outer leaves. Cut in half and set aside.

Wash the parsley in a colander under cold running water and set aside.

Wash the leeks and chop into small pieces. Set aside.

Peel the kiwis and cut in half. Set aside.

Wash the spinach thoroughly and set aside.

Now, process Brussels sprouts, parsley, leeks, kiwis, and spinach in a juicer. Transfer to serving glasses and stir in the water.

Refrigerate for 5 minutes before serving.

Nutritional information per serving: Kcal: 207, Protein: 9.8g, Carbs: 58.1g, Fats: 2.1g

7. Orange Carrot Juice

Ingredients:

1 large orange, peeled

1 large carrot, sliced

1 cup of crookneck squash, cubed

1 whole lemon, peeled

1 cup of cucumber, sliced

¼ tsp of turmeric, ground

Preparation:

Peel the orange and divide into wedges. Cut each wedge in half and set aside.

Wash and peel the carrot. Cut into thin slices and set aside.

Wash the squash and chop into small cubes. Fill the measuring cup and reserve the rest in the refrigerator. Set aside.

Peel the lemon and cut lengthwise in half. Set aside.

Wash the cucumber and cut into thin slices. Fill the measuring cup and reserve the rest for later.

Now, combine orange, carrot, squash, lemon, and cucumber in a juicer and process until juiced. Transfer to a serving glass and stir in the turmeric.

Add some crushed ice and serve immediately.

Nutrition information per serving: Kcal: 127, Protein: 4.6g, Carbs: 40.7g, Fats: 0.9g

8.   Cucumber Artichoke Juice

Ingredients:

1 cup of turnip greens

1 large cucumber

1 large artichoke head

5 large asparagus spears

Preparation:

Wash the cucumber and cut into thick slices. Set aside.

Using a sharp knife, trim off the outer leave of the artichoke. Cut into small pieces and set aside.

Wash the turnip greens and roughly chop it using hands. Set aside.

Wash the asparagus spears and trim off the woody ends. Cut into small pieces and set aside.

Now, process cucumber, artichoke, turnip greens, and asparagus in a juicer.

Transfer to serving glasses and add few ice cubes before serving.

Nutritional information per serving: Kcal: 101, Protein: 10.1g, Carbs: 35.8g, Fats: 0.8g

9.   Mango Apricot Juice

Ingredients:

1 cup of mango, chunked

3 whole apricots, chopped

1 cup of blackberries

1 cup of fresh spinach, torn

1 whole lime, peeled

Preparation:

Peel the mango and cut into small chunks. Fill the measuring cup and reserve the rest for later. Set aside.

Wash the apricots and cut in half. Remove the pits and chop into small pieces. Set aside.

Rinse the blackberries using a large colander. Drain and set aside.

Rinse the spinach thoroughly under cold running water. Drain and torn into small pieces. Set aside.

Peel the lime and cut lengthwise in half. Set aside.

Now, combine mango, apricots, blackberries, spinach, and lime in a juicer. Process until juiced. Transfer to a serving glass and refrigerate for 10 minutes before serving.

Enjoy!

Nutrition information per serving: Kcal: 201, Protein: 11.1g, Carbs: 61.5g, Fats: 2.6g

10.　Celery Mint Juice

Ingredients:

5 small celery stalks

¼ cup od fresh mint

¼ cup of fresh spinach

1 large lime, peeled

3 oz of coconut water

Preparation:

Wash the celery stalks and chop into small pieces. Set aside.

Combine mint and spinach in a large colander. Wash thoroughly under cold running water and drain. Torn into small pieces and set aside.

Peel the lime and cut in half. Set aside.

Combine lime, celery, spinach, and mint in a juicer and process until juiced.

Transfer to serving glasses and stir in coconut water. Refrigerate for 20 minutes before use.

Nutritional information per serving: Kcal: 45, Protein: 2.2g, Carbs: 16.8g, Fats: 1.6g

11.   Lemon Pepper Juice

Ingredients:

1 large lemon, peeled

½ red bell pepper, seeded

½ yellow bell pepper, seeded

1 green apple, cored

2 tbsp of chia seeds

Preparation:

Peel the lemon and cut lengthwise in half. Place it in a bowl and set aside.

Wash the bell pepper and cut in half. Remove the seeds and cut one-half of each in a bowl. Reserve the rest for some other juice.

Wash the apple and remove the core. Cut into bite-sized pieces and set aside.

Now, process lemon, bell peppers, and apple in a juicer. Transfer to serving glasses and stir in the chia seeds. Refrigerate for 15 minutes and stir again. Add some water to adjust the thickness, if needed.

Enjoy!

Nutritional information per serving: Kcal: 136, Protein: 4.3g, Carbs: 31.2g, Fats: 6.1g

12.   Pineapple Lemon Juice

Ingredients:

1 cup of pineapple, peeled

½ large lemon, peeled

1 cup of watermelon, peeled and seeded

½ tsp of ginger, ground

Preparation:

Cut the top of the pineapple using a sharp paring knife. Gently remove all hard skin and slice it into thin slices. Fill the measuring cup and reserve the rest for later.

Peel the lemon and cut lentghwise in half. Reserve one half in the refrigerator for later. Set aside.

Now, combine all ingredients in a juicer and process until juiced.

Transfer to serving glasses and add few ice cubes. Serve immediately!

Nutritional information per serving: Kcal: 41, Protein: 1.4g, Carbs: 10.2g, Fats: 0.1g

13.　　Cucumber Pear Juice

Ingredients:

2 large cucumbers

1 large pear, cored

1 cup of black grapes

1 lime, peeled

Preparation:

Wash the cucumbers and cut into thin slices. Set aside.

Wash the pear and cut in half. Remove the core and chop into bite-sized pieces. Set aside.

Wash the grapes and remove the pit. Set aside.

Peel the lime and cut lengthwise in half. Set aside.

Now, combine cucumbers, pear, grapes, and lime in a juicer and process until juiced.

Transfer to serving glasses and refrigerate for 5 minutes before serving.

Nutritional information per serving: Kcal: 113, Protein: 18.3g, Carbs: 31.3g, Fats: 0.1g

14.   Cabbage Lemon Juice

Ingredients:

1 cup of green cabbage

1 large lemon, peeled

A handful of spinach

1 medium-sized artichoke head

1 large cucumber

Preparation:

Wash the cabbage and spinach thoroughly and torn with hands. Set aside.

Peel the lemon and cut lengthwise in half. Set aside.

Using a sharp knife, trim off the outer leave of the artichoke. Cut into small pieces and set aside.

Wash the cucumber and cut into thick slices. Set aside.

Process, cabbage, lemon, spinach, cucumber, and artichoke in a juicer.

Transfer to serving glasses and add some ice.

Enjoy!

Nutritional information per serving: Kcal: 99, Protein: 8.8g, Carbs: 36.4g, Fats: 0.9g

15. Kale Lettuce Juice

Ingredients:

1 cup of fresh kale

1 cup of Romaine lettuce

1 cup of Swiss chard

1 large tomato

1 large fennel bulb

1 cup of collard greens

Preparation:

Wash the kale, lettuce, Swiss chard, and collard greens thoroughly under cold running water. Torn with hands and set aside.

Wash the tomato and chop into quarters. Set aside.

Wash the fennel bulb and trim off the wilted outer layers. Cut into small chunks and set aside.

Now, process kale, lettuce, Swiss chard, tomato, fennel and collard greens in a juicer.

Transfer to serving glasses and refrigerate for 15 minutes before serving.

Nutritional information per serving: Kcal: 106, Protein: 9.7g, Carbs: 34.8g, Fats: 1.8g

16. Artichoke Potato Juice

Ingredients:

1 large artichoke head

1 cup of sweet potatoes, cubed

1 large bunch of spinach

1 cup of turnip greens, chopped

1 cup of basil, chopped

2 oz of water

¼ tsp of Himalayan salt

Preparation:

Trim off the outer leaves of the artichoke using a sharp knife. Cut into bite-sized pieces and set aside.

Peel the sweet potato and cut into chunks. Set aside.

Combine spinach, turnip greens, and basil in a colander and wash under cold running water. Drain and chop it roughly with your hands and set aside.

Now, process artichoke, sweet potato, spinach, turnip greens, and basil in a juicer. Transfer to serving glasses and stir in the water and Himalayan salt.

Add some ice and serve immediately.

Nutritional information per serving: Kcal: 202, Protein: 18.6g, Carbs: 60.7g, Fats: 1.9g

17.   Green Lemon Apple Juice

Ingredients:

1 whole lemon, peeled

2 large green apples, cored

½ cup of fresh kale

1 large pear, cored

Preparation:

Peel the lemon and cut lengthwise in half. Set aside.

Wash the apple and cut in half. Remove the cores and chop into bite-sized pieces. Set aside.

Wash the kale thoroughly under cold running water. Drain and torn into small pieces. Set aside.

Wash the pear and cut in half. Remove the core and chop into small pieces. Set aside.

Now, combine all lemon, apples, kale, and pear in a juicer and process until juiced.

Transfer to serving glasses and add few ice cubes before serving.

Enjoy!

Nutritional information per serving: Kcal: 120, Protein: 3.2g, Carbs: 62.5g, Fats: 1.2g

18.   Broccoli Carrot Juice

Ingredients:

½ cup of fresh broccoli, chopped

3 large carrots

2 large oranges, peeled

4 collard green leaves

4 fresh kale leaves

1 garlic clove, peeled

Preparation:

Wash the broccoli thoroughly and trim off the outer layers. Chop into small pieces and reserve the rest for later. Set aside.

Wash the carrots and chop into small pieces.

Peel the oranges and divide into wedges. Set aside.

Rinse the collard greens under cold running water and drain. Torn into small pieces and set aside.

Now, combine broccoli, carrots, oranges, and collard greens in a juicer and process until juiced.

Transfer to serving glasses and serve immediately.

Nutritional information per serving: Kcal: 171, Protein: 9.2g, Carbs: 43.3g, Fats: 2.3g

19.   Broccoli Cucumber Juice

Ingredients:

1 cup of broccoli, chopped

1 large cucumber

1 cup of avocado, chopped

1 large lemon, peeled

1 large lime, peeled

1 oz of water

Preparation:

Wash the broccoli and chop into small pieces. Set aside.

Wash the cucumber and cut in thick slices. Set aside.

Peel the avocado and cut in half. Remove the pit and cut into chunks. Set aside.

Peel the lemon and lime. Cut lengthwise in half. Set aside.

Now, process broccoli, cucumber, avocado, lemon, and lime in a juicer. Transfer to serving glasses and stir in the water.

Add some ice and serve immediately.

Nutritional information per serving: Kcal: 281, Protein: 8.3g, Carbs: 38.8g, Fats: 22.8g

20.   Beet Turmeric Juice

Ingredients:

1 cup of beet greens, torn

¼ tsp of turmeric powder, ground

2 cups of parsley, torn

1 whole cucumber, sliced

1 cup of celery, chopped

1 whole leek, chopped

¼ tsp of cumin, ground

Preparation:

Combine beet greens and parsley in a large colander. Rinse well under cold running water and drain. Torn into small pieces and set aside.

Wash the cucumber and cut into thin slices. Set aside.

Wash the celery and chop into small pieces. Fill the measuring cup and reserve the rest in the refrigerator. Set aside.

Wash the leek and chop into bite-sized pieces. Set aside.

Now, combine parsley, beet greens, cucumber, celery, and leek in a juicer and process until juiced. Transfer to a serving glass and stir in the turmeric and cumin.

Serve immediately.

Nutrition information per serving: Kcal: 127, Protein: 8.4g, Carbs: 35.7g, Fats: 1.7g

21.   Cucumber Pineapple Juice

Ingredients:

1 large cucumber

1 cup of pineapple, chopped

3 celery stalks

½ cup of fresh spinach

¼ tsp of ginger, ground

¼ tsp of turmeric, ground

Preparation:

Wash the cucumber and cut into thin slices. Set aside.

Cut the top of the pineapple using a sharp paring knife. Gently remove all hard skin and slice it into thin slices. Fill the measuring cup and reserve the rest for later.

Wash the celery and cut into small pieces. Set aside.

Rinse the spinach thoroughly under cold running water and drain. Torn into small pieces and set aside.

Now, combine cucumber, pineapple, celery, and spinach in a juicer and process until juiced.

Transfer to serving glasses and stir in the turmeric and ginger.

Serve immediately.

Nutritional information per serving: Kcal: 109, Protein: 3.3g, Carbs: 61.2g, Fats: 1.3g

22. Orange Cucumber Juice

Ingredients:

1 cup of broccoli, chopped

2 large oranges, peeled

1 large cucumber, peeled

1 large carrot

Preparation:

Wash the broccoli and trim off the outer leaves. Cut into small pieces and fill the measuring cup. Reserve the rest in the refrigerator.

Peel the oranges and divide into wedges. Set aside.

Wash the cucumber and cut into thin slices. Set aside.

Now, combine broccoli, oranges, cucumber, and carrot in a juicer and process until juiced.

Transfer to serving glasses and add few ice cubes.

Serve immediately!

Nutritional information per serving: Kcal: 68, Protein: 2.3g, Carbs: 19.7g, Fats: 0.1g

23. Apple Ginger Juice

Ingredients:

1 large Granny Smith's apple, cored and chopped

1 small ginger knob, peeled

1 cup of celery, chopped

1 cup of fresh mint, torn

¼ tsp of liquid honey

1 oz of water

Preparation:

Wash the apple and cut lengthwise in half. Remove the core and cut into bite-sized pieces. Set aside.

Peel the ginger knob and chop into small pieces. Set aside.

Wash the celery and chop into small pieces. Fill the measuring cup and reserve the rest for later.

Rinse the mint thoroughly under cold running water. Dran and torn into small pieces.

Now, combine apple, ginger, celery, and mint in a juicer and process until well juiced. Transfer to a serving glass and stir in the honey and water.

Refrigerate for 5 minutes before serving.

Enjoy!

Nutrition information per serving: Kcal: 121, Protein: 2.6g, Carbs: 35.8g, Fats: 0.8g

24.   Spring Onion Pepper Juice

Ingredients:

1 medium-sized spring onion

1 large bell pepper, seeded

1 cup of cherry tomatoes

1 garlic clove, peeled

¼ tsp of Cayenne pepper, ground

¼ tsp of salt

A handful of fresh cilantro

Preparation:

Wash the spring onion and chop into small pieces. Set aside.

Wash the bell pepper and cut in half. Remove the seeds and chop into small pieces. Set aside.

Wash the cilantro thoroughly and torn with hands. Set aside.

Wash the cherry tomatoes and place them in a bowl. Cut in half and reserve the juice while cutting. Set aside.

Peel the garlic and set aside.

Now, process spring onion, bell pepper, cilantro, tomatoes, and garlic in a juicer.

Transfer to serving glasses and stir in Cayenne pepper and salt.

Refrigerate for 5 minutes and serve.

Nutritional information per serving: Kcal: 41, Protein: 2.8g, Carbs: 11.5g, Fats: 0.6g

25. Grape Apple Juice

Ingredients:

1 cup of green grapes

1 Granny Smith apple, cored

3 large carrots

1 large lemon, peeled

A handful of spinach

2 oz of water

Preparation:

Wash the grapes and set aside.

Wash the apple and remove the core. Cut into bite-sized pieces and set aside.

Wash the carrots and cut into thick slices. Set aside.

Peel the lemon and cut lengthwise in half. Set aside.

Wash the spinach thoroughly under cold running water. Roughly chop it and set aside.

Now, combine grapes, apple, carrots, lemon, and spinach in a juicer and process until juiced. Transfer to serving glasses and stir in the water.

Refrigerate for 10 minutes before serving.

Enjoy!

Nutritional information per serving: Kcal: 208, Protein: 1.4g, Carbs: 62.6g, Fats: 1.4g

26.   Broccoli Carrot Juice

Ingredients:

1 cup of fresh broccoli

4 large carrots

1 large green apple, cored

1 tsp of ginger root

2 cups of cauliflower, chopped

Preparation:

Wash the broccoli and trim off the outer leaves. Cut into small pieces and fill the measuring cups. Reserve the rest in the refrigerator.

Wash the carrots and cut into thin slices. Set aside.

Wash the apple and cut in half. Remove the core and cut into bite-sized pieces. Set aside.

Peel the ginger root and set aside.

Wash the cauliflower and trim off the outer leaves. Chop into small pieces and set aside.

Now, combine broccoli, carrots, apple, ginger, and cauliflower in a juicer and process until juiced.

Transfer to serving glasses and optionally, garnish with mint.

Enjoy!

Nutritional information per serving: Kcal: 136, Protein: 6.3g, Carbs: 42.8g, Fats: 1.2g

27.   Apple Spinach Juice

Ingredients:

1 large apple, cored

1 cup of fresh spinach

1 tbsp of chia seeds

¼ tsp of cinnamon, ground

Preparation:

Wash the apple and cut in half. Remove the core and cut into bite-sized pieces. Set aside.

Wash the spinach thoroughly under cold running water.Drain and torn into small pieces. Set aside.

Now, combine apple, spinach, and chia in a juicer and process until juiced.

Transfer to serving glasses and stir in the cinnamon.

Refrigerate for 10 minutes and serve.

Nutritional information per serving: Kcal: 121, Protein: 4.3g, Carbs: 27.8g, Fats: 5.3g

28.   Pear Carrot Juice

Ingredients:

1 large pear, cored

3 large carrots

1 medium-sized cucumber

1 large lemon, peeled

¼ cup of fresh mint

½ cup of broccoli

½ tsp of ginger, ground

½ tsp of green tea powder

2 oz of water

Preparation:

Wash the pear and cut in half. Remove the core and chop into small pieces. Set aside.

Wash the carrots and cucumber. Cut into thin slices and set aside.

Peel the lemon and cut lengthwise in half. Set aside.

Combine pear, carrots, cucumber, lemon, mint, ginger,

and broccoli in a juicer and process until juiced.

Mix water with green tea in a serving glasses and add juice.

Mix with a spoon and add few ice cubes. Serve immediately.

Nutritional information per serving: Kcal: 141, Protein: 5.5g, Carbs: 45.7g, Fats: 0.9g

29.   Watercress Pumpkin Juice

Ingredients:

1 cup of watercress, chopped

1 cup of pumpkin, chopped

1 cup of cherry tomatoes, halved

1 cup of collard greens, chopped

1 large cucumber

Preparation:

Combine watercress and collard greens in a colander and wash thoroughly. Torn with hands and set aside.

Peel the pumpkin and cut in half. Scoop out the seeds using a spoon. Cut one large wedge and peel it. Cut into small chunks and set aside. Reserve the rest for later.

Wash the tomatoes and place them in a bowl. Cut in half and reserve the juice in the bowl while cutting. Set aside.

Wash the cucumber and cut into thick slices. Set aside.

Now, process watercress, collard greens, pumpkin, tomatoes, and cucumber in a juicer. Transfer to serving glasses and stir in the reserved tomato juice. Add some ice before serving.

Enjoy!

Nutritional information per serving: Kcal: 96, Protein: 6.4g, Carbs: 27.4g, Fats: 1g

30.   Zucchini Asparagus Juice

Ingredients:

2 medium-sized zucchini, sliced

6 medium asparagus stalks, trimmed and chopped

3 Roma tomatoes, chopped

4 large carrots, sliced

Preparation:

Wash the zucchini and cut into thin slices. Set aside.

Wash the asparagus and trim off the woody ends. cut into small pieces. Set aside.

Wash the tomatoes and cut into small pieces. Make sure to reserve the juices while cutting.

Wash the carrots and cut into thin slices. Set aside.

Now, combine all ingredients in a juicer and process until juiced.

Transfer to serving glasses and enjoy immediately.

Nutritional information per serving: Kcal: 92, Protein: 5.4g, Carbs: 27.3g, Fats: 0.9g

31.   Celery Apple Juice

Ingredients:

3 celery stalks

1 large green apple, cored

1 large lemon, peeled

½ cup of cilantro

½ tsp of ginger, ground

Preparation:

Wash the celery and chop into small pieces. Set aside.

Wash the apple and cut in half. Remove the core and cut into small pieces. Set aside.

Peel the lemon and cut lengthwise in half. Set aside.

Now, combine celery, apple, lemon, and cilantro in a juicer. Process until juiced. Transfer to serving glasses and stir in the ginger.

Add few ice cubes and serve immediately.

Nutritional information per serving: Kcal: 73, Protein: 2.2g, Carbs: 26.7g, Fats: 0.1g

32.   Chia Carrot Juice

Ingredients:

3 large carrots

2 large apples, cored

½ tsp of ginger, ground

1 tbsp of chia seeds

Preparation:

Wash the carrots and cut into thin slices. Set aside.

Wash the apples and cut in half. Remove the core and cut into bite-sized pieces. Set aside.

Now, combine carrots, apples, and ginger in a juicer and process until juiced.

Transfer to serving glasses and stir in the chia seeds. Add few ice cubes and enjoy!

Nutritional information per serving: Kcal: 177, Protein: 3.2g, Carbs: 28.4g, Fats: 4.6g

33. Kale Apple Juice

Ingredients:

1 medium fennel

½ cup of fresh kale

1 large green apple, cored

4 tangerines, peeled

Preparation:

Wash the kale thoroughly under cold running water. Drain and set aside.

Wash the apple and cut in half. Remove the core and cut into bite-sized pieces. Set aside.

Peel the tangerines and divide into wedges. Set aside.

Trim off the outside layers of the fennel. Wash it and cut into bite-sized pieces. Set aside.

Now, combine kale, apple, tangerines, and fennel in a juicer and process until juiced.

Transfer to serving glasses and add few ice cubes or refrigerate before use.

Nutritional information per serving: Kcal: 121, Protein: 4.3g, Carbs: 31.3g, Fats: 1.3g

34.   Lime Cucumber Juice

Ingredients:

1 large lime, peeled

1 large cucumber

½ cup of fresh kale

1 celery stalk

1 small jalapeno pepper, seeded

Preparation:

Peel the lime and cut lengthwise in half. Set aside.

Wash the cucumber and cut into thin slices. Set aside.

Rinse the kale thoroughly under cold running water. Drain and set aside.

Wash the celery and chop it into small pieces. Set aside.

Now, combine lime, cucumber, kale, and celery in a juicer and process until juiced. Add coconut water if it is too spicy.

Transfer to serving glasses and add a few ice cubes.

Serve immediately.

Nutritional information per serving: Kcal: 171, Protein: 3.2g, Carbs: 47.3g, Fats: 1.3g

35.   Pomegranate Pumpkin Juice

Ingredients:

1 cup of pomegranate seeds

1 cup of pumpkin, cubed

1 medium-sized orange, peeled

3 whole plums, pitted and chopped

¼ tsp of ginger, ground

1 oz of water

Preparation:

Cut the top of the pomegranate fruit using a sharp paring knife. Slice down to each of the white membranes inside of the fruit. Pop the seeds into a measuring cup and set aside.

Cut the top of a pumpkin. Cut lengthwise in half and then scrape out the seeds. Cut one large wedge and peel it. Cut into small cubes and fill the measuring cup. Reserve the rest in the refrigerator.

Wash the plums and cut into halves. Remove the pits and chop into small pieces.Set aside.

Peel the orange and divide into wedges. Cut each wedge in half and set aside.

Now, combine pomegranate, pumpkin, plums, and orange in a juicer. Process until juiced. Transfer to a serving glass and stir in the ginger and water.

Refrigerate for 5 minutes before serving.

Enjoy!

Nutrition information per serving: Kcal: 214, Protein: 5.2g, Carbs: 61.8g, Fats: 1.8g

36.   Kiwi Cucumber Juice

Ingredients:

2 kiwis, peeled

1 large cucumber

1 cup of fresh strawberries

1 whole lime, peeled

2 tbsp of fresh mint

Preparation:

Peel the kiwis and cut in half. Set aside.

Wash the cucumber and cut into thin slices. Set aside.

Wash the strawberries and remove the top stems, if any. Cut into small pieces and set aside.

Peel the lime and cut lengthwise in half. Set aside.

Now, combine kiwis, cucumber, strawberries, lime and mint in a juicer and process until juiced.

Transfer to serving glasses and refrigerate for a while until use.

Nutritional information per serving: Kcal: 91, Protein: 3.1g, Carbs: 29.9g, Fats: 0.9g

37.   Beet Fennel Juice

Ingredients:

1 cup of beets, chopped

1 cup of fennel, sliced

2 large tomatoes, peeled

1 tbsp of fresh mint, chopped

1 cup of red leaf lettuce, shredded

½ tsp of ginger, ground

Preparation:

Wash the beets and trim off the green ends. Cut into small pieces and set aside.

Wash the fennel bulb and trim off the wilted outer layers. Cut into small chunks and set aside.

Wash the tomatoes and place them in a bowl. Cut into quarters and reserve the juice while cutting.

Wash the lettuce thoroughly and torn with hands. Set aside.

Now, combine beets, fennel, tomatoes, mint, and lettuce in a juicer and process until juiced.

Transfer to serving glasses and stir in the ground ginger.

Refrigerate for 10 minutes before serving.

Nutritional information per serving: Kcal: 111, Protein: 6.9g, Carbs: 34.8g, Fats: 1.2g

38.   Celery Kale Juice

Ingredients:

1 cup of celery, chopped

1 cup of fresh kale, torn

1 cup of asparagus, trimmed

1 cup of mustard greens, torn

1 large lemon

1 large cucumber

Preparation:

Wash the celery thoroughly and cut into bite-sized pieces. Set aside.

Combine kale and mustard greens in a colander and wash under cold running water. Torn with hands and set aside.

Wash the asparagus and trim off the woody ends. Cut into small pieces and set aside.

Peel the lemon and cut lengthwise in half. Set aside.

Wash the cucumber and cut into thick slices. Set aside.

Now, process celery, kale, asparagus, mustard greens,

lemon, and cucumber in a juicer.

Transfer to serving glasses and add few ice cubes before serving.

Enjoy!

Nutritional information per serving: Kcal: 107, Protein: 10.7g, Carbs: 33g, Fats: 1.7g

39.   Parsley Apple Juice

Ingredients:

2 tbsp of fresh parsley

2 large apples, cored

2 large carrots

½ cup of fresh spinach

¼ tsp of ginger, ground

1 tbsp of flaxseeds

Preparation:

Combine parsley and spinach in a large colander. Wash under cold running water. Drain and torn into small pieces. Set aside.

Wash the apples and cut in half. Remove the core and cut into bite-size pieces. Set aside.

Wash the carrots and cut into thin slices. Set aside.

Now, combine parsley, apples, spinach, and carrots in a juicer. Process until juiced. Transfer to serving glasses and stir in the ginger and flaxseeds.

Add few ice cubes and serve!

Nutritional information per serving: Kcal: 119, Protein: 4.3g, Carbs: 62.2g, Fats: 2.3g

40.   Zucchini Carrot Juice

Ingredients:

1 medium-sized zucchini, chunked

1 large carrot, sliced

1 large artichoke

1 red leaf lettuce, torn

1 cup of watercress, torn

3 oz of water

Preparation:

Peel the zucchini and cut in half. Scoop out the seeds and cut into chunks. Set aside. Set aside.

Wash the carrot and cut into thick slices. Set aside.

Trim off the outer leaves of the artichoke using a sharp knife. Cut into small pieces and set aside.

Combine red leaf lettuce and watercress in a colander. Wash under cold running water. Drain and torn with hands. Set aside.

Now, process zucchini, carrot, artichoke, red leaf lettuce, and watercress in a juicer. Transfer to serving glasses and stir in the water.

You can sprinkle with some fresh mint, but this is optional.

Add few ice cubes and serve immediately.

Nutritional information per serving: Kcal: 94, Protein: 9.4g, Carbs: 31.1g, Fats: 1.1g

41.   Kale Squash Juice

Ingredients:

¼ cup of fresh kale

½ yellow squash, peeled and chopped

1 medium-sized broccoli

1 large apple, cored

¼ cup of fresh spinach

4 small carrots, sliced

Preparation:

Combine kale and spinach in a large colander. Rinse under cold running water and torn into small pieces. Set aside.

Peel the squash and cut in half. Scoop out the seeds and chop into small pieces. Reserve the rest in the refrigerator.

Wash the broccoli and chop into small pieces. Set aside.

Wash the apple and cut in half. Remove the core and chop into small pieces. Set aside.

Wash and peel the carrot. Cut into small slices and set aside.

Now, combine kale, spinach, squash, broccoli, apple, and carrot in a juicer. Process until well juiced. Transfer to a serving glasses and add few ice cubes.

Serve immediately.

Nutritional information per serving: Kcal: 81, Protein: 2.3g, Carbs: 18.4g, Fats: 0.2g

42.   Strawberry Apple Juice

Ingredients:

1 cup of strawberries

1 large green apple, cored

3 large peaches, pitted

¼ tsp of cinnamon, ground

Preparation:

Wash the strawberries and remove the top stem. Chop into small pieces and fill the measuring cup. Reserve the rest in the refrigerator.

Wash the apple and cut in half. Remove the core and chop into bite-sized pieces. Set aside.

Wash the peaches and cut in half. Remove the pits and chop into small pieces. Set aside.

Now, combine strawberries, apple, and peaches in a juicer. Process until juiced. Transfer to a serving glass and stir in the cinnamon.

Refrigerate for 10 minutes before serving.

Nutritional information per serving: Kcal: 64, Protein: 1.2g, Carbs: 18.3g, Fats: 0.1g

43.   Blueberry Grapefruit Juice

Ingredients:

1 cup of blueberries

1 whole grapefruit, peeled

1 cup of avocado, cubed

1 small Red Delicious apple, cored

1 tsp of peppermint extract

Preparation:

Place the blueberries in a colander. Rinse well under cold running water and drain. Set aside.

Peel the grapefruit and divide into wedges. Cut each wedge in half and set aside.

Peel the avocado and cut lengthwise in half. Remove the pit and cut into small cubes. Fill the measuring cup and reserve the rest in the refrigerator.

Wash the apple and cut lengthwise in half. Remove the core and cut into bite-sized pieces. Set aside.

Now, combine blueberries, grapefruit, avocado, and apple in a juicer and process until juiced. Transfer to a serving glass and stir in the peppermint extract.

Refrigerate for 5 minutes before serving.

Nutrition information per serving: Kcal: 436, Protein: 6.4g, Carbs: 69.5g, Fats: 23.2g

44.   Lemon Papaya Juice

Ingredients:

1 large lemon, peeled and halved

1 cup of papaya, chopped

1 large green apple, cored

1 cup of cantaloupe, cubed

1 large cucumber

Preparation:

Peel the lemon and cut lengthwise in half. Set aside.

Peel the papaya and cut lengthwise in half. Scoop out the black seeds and flesh using a spoon. Cut into small chunks and fill the measuring cup. Refrigerate the rest for some other juice recipe. Set aside.

Wash the apple and remove the core. Cut into bite-sized pieces and set aside.

Cut the cantaloupe in half. Scoop out the seeds and flesh. Cut two wedges and peel them. Chop into chunks and set aside. Reserve the rest of the cantaloupe in a refrigerator.

Wash the cucumber and cut into thick slices. Set aside.

Now, process lemon, papaya, apple, cantaloupe, and cucumber in a juicer. Transfer to serving glasses and add few ice cubes before serving.

Enjoy!

Nutritional information per serving: Kcal: 245, Protein: 5.5g, Carbs: 72.8g, Fats: 1.6g

45.   Kale Apple Juice

Ingredients:

½ cup of fresh kale

1 large green apple, cored

½ cup of pomegranate seeds

¼ tsp of ginger, ground

3-4 fresh mint leaves

Preparation:

Rinse the kale thoroughly under cold running water. Drain well and torn into small pieces. Set aside.

Wash the apple and cut in half. Remove the core and cut into bite-sized pieces. Set aside.

Cut the top of the pomegranate fruit using a sharp knife. Slice down to each of the white membranes inside of the fruit. Pop the seeds into a small bowl. Set aside.

Now, combine kale, apple, and pomegranate seeds in a juicer and process until juiced. Transfer to serving glasses and stir in the ginger.

Add few ice cubes and top with mint leaves. Add few ice

cubes and serve immediately.

Nutritional information per serving: Kcal: 143, Protein: 6.2g, Carbs: 41.2g, Fats: 2.4g

46.   Orange Coconut Juice

Ingredients:

1 large orange, peeled

1 tsp of pure coconut sugar

½ cup of butternut squash, chunked

2 slices of fresh ginger

1 large red delicious apple, peeled and cored

1 large carrot, sliced

Preparation:

Peel the orange and divide into wedges. Set aside.

Peel the ginger slices and cut into small pieces. Set aside.

Combine 2 tablespoons of water and coconut sugar in a small bowl. Stir well let it stand for 5 minutes, or until sugar completely disolved.

Peel the butternut squash and remove the seeds using a spoon. Cut into small cubes and reserve the rest of the squash for some other recipe. Wrap in a plastic foil and refrigerate.

Wash the apple and remove the core. Cut into bite-sized

pieces and set aside.

Wash the carrot and cut into small slices. Set aside.

Now, process orange, ginger, butternut squash, apple, carrot, and in a juicer. Transfer to serving glasses and stir in the coconut mixture.

Add few ice cubes and serve immediately.

Nutritional information per serving: Kcal: 314, Protein: 5.3g, Carbs: 61g, Fats: 1.2g

47.   Italian Vegetable Juice

Ingredients:

3 large cucumbers

1 large bell pepper, seeded

2 large tomatoes, halved

2 garlic cloves, peeled

1 large lime, peeled

¼ cup of fresh cilantro

Preparation:

Wash the cucumber and chop into thin slices. Set aside.

Wash the bell pepper and cut in half. Remove the seeds and chop into small pieces. Set aside.

Wash the tomatoes and chop into small pieces. Make sure to reserve the tomato juice while cutting. Set aside.

Peel the lime and cut in half. Set aside.

Wash the cilantro and chop into small pieces. Set aside.

Now, combine cucumber, bell pepper, tomatoes, lime, and cilantro in a juicer. Process until juiced. Transfer to a serving glass and serve immediately.

Nutritional information per serving: Kcal: 109, Protein: 6.4g, Carbs: 38.5g, Fats: 1.2g

48.　　Carrot Cucumber Juice

Ingredients:

1 large carrot

1 large cucumber

1 cup of butternut squash, chopped

1 large guava

1 large orange

1 tbsp of honey

Preparation:

Wash the carrot and cut into thin slices. Set aside.

Peel the cucumber and cut into thin slices. Set aside.

Peel the butternut squash and remove the seeds using a spoon. Cut into small cubes and reserve the rest of the squash for some other recipe. Wrap in a plastic foil and refrigerate.

Peel the guava and cut into chunks. Set aside.

Now, combine, carrot, cucumber, butternut squash, guava, and orange in a juicer and process until juiced.

Transfer to serving glasses and stir in the honey.

Add some ice and serve immediately.

Nutritional information per serving: Kcal: 266, Protein: 7.2g, Carbs: 80.7g, Fats: 1.4g

49.   Lemon Banana Juice

Ingredients:

1 whole lemon, peeled

1 large banana, chunked

1 cup of strawberries, chopped

1 cup of pineapple, chunked

1 tbsp of fresh mint, finely chopped

Preparation:

Peel the lemon and cut lengthwise in half. Set aside.

Peel the banana and cut into small chunks. Set aside.

Wash the strawberries and remove the stems. Chop into small pieces and fill the measuring cup. Reserve the rest in the refrigerator.

Cut the top of the pineapple using a sharp paring knife. Gently remove all hard skin and slice it into thin slices. Fill the measuring cup and reserve the rest for later.

Now, combine lemon, banana, strawberries, and pineapple in a juicer. Process until juiced. Transfer to a serving glass and stir in the mint.

Add few ice cubes and serve immediately.

Nutrition information per serving: Kcal: 224, Protein: 4.1g, Carbs: 69.4g, Fats: 1.3g

50.   Pepper Basil Juice

Ingredients:

2 large red bell peppers, chopped

1 cup of fresh basil, torn

3 large beets, trimmed

1 large lime,peeled and halved

1 cup of red leaf lettuce, torn

 1 large cucumber

Preparation:

Wash the red bell peppers and cut in half. Remove the seeds and roughly chop it. Set aside.

Wash the beets and trim off the green parts. Cut into small pieces and set aside.

Peel the lime and cut lengthwise in half. Set aside.

Combine basila and red leaf lettuce in a large colander and wash thoroughly under cold running water. Drain and torn into small pieces. Set aside.

Wash the cucumber and cut into thin slices. Set aside.

Now, process red bell peppers, basil, beets, lime, red leaf lettuce, and cucumber in a juicer. Transfer to serving glasses and add few ice cubes.

Serve immediately.

Nutritional information per serving: Kcal: 208, Protein: 10.5g, Carbs: 59.2g, Fats: 1.9g

51. Basil Lime Juice

Ingredients:

½ cup of fresh basil

1 large lime, peeled

½ cup of Swiss chard

2 large green apples, cored

¼ cup of fresh mint

Preparation:

Combine basil, Swiss chard, and mint in a large colander and rinse under cold running water. Drain and torn into small pieces. Set aside.

Peel the lime and cut lengthwise in half. Set aside.

Wash the apples and cut in half. Remove the core and cut into bite-sized pieces. Set aside.

Now, combine basil, Swiss chard, mint, lime, and apples in a juicer. Process until well juiced.

Transfer to serving glasses and add few ice cubes or refrigerate until use.

Nutritional information per serving: Kcal: 114, Protein: 2.3g, Carbs: 30.4g, Fats: 0.2g

52.   Radish Beet Juice

Ingredients:

3 large radishes, chopped

2 cups of beet greens, torn

2 large leeks, chopped

1 cup of collard greens, torn

1 large cucumber

½ tsp of Himalayan salt

¼ tsp of Cayenne pepper, ground

3 oz of water

Preparation:

Wash the radishes and trim off the green parts. Cut in half and set aside.

Combine beet greens and collard greens in a colander. Wash thoroughly under cold running water. Drain and set aside.

Wash the leeks and chop into small pieces. Set aside.

Wash the cucumber and cut into thick slices. Set aside-

Now, combine radishes, beet greens, leeks, collard greens, and cucumber in a juicer and process until juiced.

Transfer to serving glasses and stir in the salt, Cayenne pepper, and water.

Refrigerate for 10 minutes before serving.

Enjoy!

Nutritional information per serving: Kcal: 148, Protein: 7.6g, Carbs: 42.3g, Fats: 1.2g

53.   Carrot Watercress Juice

Ingredients:

2 large carrots, sliced

½ cup of watercress, torn

1 cup of pineapple, chunked

1 large lemon, peeled

¼ tsp of fresh ginger root, ground

Preparation:

Wash and peel the carrots. Cut into thin slices and set aside.

Rinse the watercress under cold running water. Drain well and torn into small pieces. Fill the measuring cup and reserve the rest for later.

Cut the top of a pineapple and peel it using a sharp knife. Cut into small chunks and fill the measuring cup. Reserve the rest of the pineapple in a refrigerator.

Peel the lemon and cut lengthwise in half. Set aside.

Now, combine carrots, watercress, pineapple, and lemon in a juicer. Process until juiced. Transfer to a serving glass and stir in the ginger.

Add some ice and serve.

Nutritional information per serving: Kcal: 101, Protein: 3.1g, Carbs: 34.2g, Fats: 1.1g

54. Pineapple Orange Juice

Ingredients:

1 cup of pineapple chunks

1 large orange, peeled and wedged

1 cup of avocado, cubed

1 large cucumber, sliced

2 oz of water

Preparation:

Cut the top of a pineapple and peel it using a sharp knife. Cut into small chunks. Reserve the rest of the pineapple in a refrigerator.

Peel the orange and divide into wedges. Set aside.

Peel the avocado and cut in half. Remove the pit and cut into small cubes. Fill the measuring cup and reserve the rest in the refrigerator.

Wash the cucumber and cut into thick slices. Set aside.

Now, combine pineapple, orange, avocado, and cucumber in a juicer and process until juiced.

Transfer to serving glasses and stir in the water. Add few

ice cubes and serve immediately.

Nutritional information per serving: Kcal: 375, Protein: 7.5g, Carbs: 66.6g, Fats: 22.15g

55. Tomato Mustard Green Juice

Ingredients:

1 medium-sized Roma tomato, chopped

1 cup of mustard greens, torn

2 cups of Romaine lettuce, chopped

1 cup of parsley, torn

1 whole cucumber, sliced

¼ tsp of turmeric, ground

¼ tsp of salt

Preparation:

Wash the tomato and place in a bowl. Chop into bite-sized pieces and reserve the tomato juice while cutting. Set aside.

Combine mustard greens, lettuce, and parsley in a large colander. Rinse well and drain. Torn into small pieces and set aside.

Wash the cucumber and cut into thin slices. Set aside.

Now, combine tomato, mustard greens, lettuce, parsley, and cucumber in a juicer and process until juiced. Transfer to a serving glass and stir in the turmeric, salt, and reserved tomato juice.

Refrigerate for 5 minutes before serving.

Enjoy!

Nutrition information per serving: Kcal: 85, Protein: 7.6g, Carbs: 25.3g, Fats: 1.6g

56.   Peach Pomegranate Juice

Ingredients:

2 large peaches, pitted

1 cup of pomegranate seeds

5 large plums, pitted

1 large carrot

Preparation:

Wash the plums and peaches and cut in half. Remove the pits and set aside.

Cut the top of the pomegranate fruit using a sharp knife. Slice down to each of the white membranes inside of the fruit. Pop the seeds into a small bowl. Set aside.

Wash the carrot and cut into small pieces. Set aside.

Now, combine plums, peaches, pomegranate seeds, and carrot in a juicer and process until juiced.

Transfer to serving glasses and refrigerate for 10 minutes before serving.

Nutritional information per serving: Kcal: 326, Protein: 7.6g, Carbs: 94.2g, Fats: 3.1g

57.   Beet Lime Juice

Ingredients:

1 small cauliflower head, chopped

2 large beets, trimmed

1 large lime, peeled and halved

2 large radishes, chopped

¼ tsp of Himalayan salt

3 oz of water

Preparation:

Wash the beets and radishes. Trim off the green parts and cut into bite-sized pieces. Set aside.

Peel the lime and cut lengthwise in half. Set aside.

Trim off the outer leaves of cauliflower. Wash it and cut into small pieces. Set aside.

Now, combine beets, lime, cauliflower, and radishes in a juicer. Transfer to serving glasses and stir in the salt and water.

Add some ice cubes and serve immediately.

Nutritional information per serving: Kcal: 135, Protein: 9.3g, Carbs: 41g, Fats: 1.2g

58.   Melon Apple Juice

Ingredients:

1 large wedge of honeydew melon

1 small Grany Smith's apple, cored

2 cups of blueberries

1 oz of coconut water

1 tsp of vanilla extract

1 tbsp of mint, finely chopped

Preparation:

Cut melon lengthwise in half. Scoop out the seeds and then wash. Cut one large wedge and peel it. Cut into small cubes and set aside.

Wash the apple and cut lengthwise in half. Remove the core and cut into bite-sized pieces. Set aside.

Place the blueberries in a large colander. Rinse well under cold running water and drain. Set aside.

Now, combine honeydew melon, apple, and blueberries in a juicer. Process until juiced.

Transfer to a serving glass and stir in the coconut water,

vanilla extract, and mint. Add some crushed ice and serve immediately.

Nutrition information per serving: Kcal: 263, Protein: 3.7g, Carbs: 77.1g, Fats: 1.5g

59.   Grapefruit Rosemary Juice

Ingredients:

3 large grapefruits, peeled

3 large oranges, peeled

1 large lemon, peeled

½ tsp of fresh rosemary

Preparation:

Peel the grapefruit and oranges. Cut into bite-sized pieces. Set aside.

Peel the lemon and cut lengthwise in half. Set aside.

Combine all ingredients in a juicer and process until juiced. Transfer to serving glasses and add few ice cubes.

Sprinkle with fresh rosemary and serve immediately!

Nutritional information per serving: Kcal: 140, Protein: 3.4g, Carbs: 37.6g, Fats: 0.1g

60.   Carrot Lemon Juice

Ingredients:

3 large carrots

1 large lemon, peeled

1 cup of green beans

1 cup of fresh kale, torn

1 large cucumber

1 tbsp of honey, raw

Preparation:

Wash the carrots and cut into thick slices. Set aside.

Peel the lemon and cut lengthwise in half. Set aside.

Wash the kale thoroughly under cold running water. Drain and set aside.

Wash the green beans and place them in a medium pot. Add water enough to cover and soak for at least 2 hours. Set aside.

Now, process carrots, lemon, green beans, kale, and cucumber in a juicer.

Transfer to serving glasses and stir in the honey. Refrigerate for 5 minutes and serve.

Enjoy!

Nutritional information per serving: Kcal: 239, Protein: 9.4g, Carbs: 50g, Fats: 1.8g

61.   Lime Beet Juice

Ingredients:

2 large limes, peeled

1 cup of beet greens, torn

2 large cucumbers, peeled

1 cup of kale, chopped

1 cup of parsley, chopped

1 tbsp of agave syrup

½ cup of pure coconut water, unsweetened

Preparation:

Peel the limes and cut into quarters and add to the bowl.

Wash the beet greens and torn into a bowl with other ingredients.

Wash the cucumbers and cut into thick slices. Place them in a medium bowl and set aside.

Combine parsley and kale in a colander and wash with cold running water. Roughly chop it and add to the bowl.

Now, process limes, beet greens, cucumber, kale, and

parsley in a juicer. Transfer to serving glasses and stir in the agave syrup and coconut water.

Add some ice and serve immediately.

Nutritional information per serving: Kcal: 139, Protein: 10.6g, Carbs: 42.2g, Fats: 1.9g

62.   Apple Orange Juice

Ingredients:

1 medium-sized red apple, cored

1 large orange, peeled

2 large peaches, chopped

1 ginger root knob, 1-inch

2 oz of water

Preparation:

Wash the apple and remove the core. Cut into bite-sized pieces and set aside.

Peel the orange and divide into wedges. Set aside.

Wash the peaches and cut in half. Remove the pits and cut into small pieces. Set aside.

Peel the ginger root knob and set aside.

Now, process apple, orange, peaches, and ginger in a juicer. Transfer to serving glasses and stir in the water.

Add some ice or refrigerate before serving.

Nutritional information per serving: Kcal: 294, Protein: 5.6g, Carbs: 85.8g, Fats: 1.5g

63.   Asparagus Broccoli Juice

Ingredients:

4 medium-sized asparagus spears, trimmed

1 large broccoli

1 large green apple, cored

3 large celery stalks

A handful of fresh parsley

Preparation:

Wash the asparagus and trim off the woody ends. Cut into small pieces and set aside.

Wash the celery stalks and broccoli. Chop into small pieces. Set aside.

Wash the apple and remove the core. Cut into bite-sized pieces and set aside.

Wash the parsley and finely chop it. Place it in a small bowl and add olive oil. Let it stand for 5 minutes.

Now, process asparagus, broccoli, apple, and celery in a juicer. Transfer to serving glasses and stir in the parsley and oil. You can sprinkle with some salt to taste if you like, but this is optional.

Serve immediately.

Nutritional information per serving: Kcal: 134, Protein: 7.3g, Carbs: 45.9g, Fats: 1.7g

64.   Mango Apple Juice

Ingredients:

1 cup of mango chunks

1 medium-sized green apple, cored

1 cup of cranberries

1 large honeydew melon wedge, chopped

1 cup of fresh mint

½ cup of hot water

Preparation:

Peel the mango and cut into chunks. Set aside.

Wash the apple and remove the core. Cut into bite-sized pieces and set aside.

Place the cranberries in a colander and wash under cold running water. Drain and set aside.

Cut the honeydew melon lengthwise in half. Scoop out the seeds using a spoon. Cut the large wedges and peel them. Cut into small chunks and place in a bowl. Wrap the rest of the melon in a plastic foil and refrigerate.

Combine mint with hot water and let it stand for 5

minutes.

Now, process mango, apple, cranberries, honeydew melon, and mint in a juicer. Transfer to serving glasses and add water from the soaked mint. Refrigerate for 5 minutes before serving.

Nutritional information per serving: Kcal: 261, Protein: 4.3g, Carbs: 79.1g, Fats: 1.5g

65. Blueberry Basil Juice

Ingredients:

1 cup of blackberries

1 cup of blueberries

1 cup of fresh basil

1 large beet, trimmed

2 oz of coconut water

Preparation:

Combine blackberries and blueberries in a colander and wash under cold running water. Set aside.

Wash the basil thoroughly and roughly chop it using hands.

Wash the beet and trim off the green ends. Chop into small pieces and set aside.

Now, combine blueberries, basil, blackberries, and beet in a juicer and process until juiced.

Transfer to serving glasses and stir in the coconut water.

Add some ice and serve immediately.

Nutritional information per serving: Kcal: 142, Protein: 5.2g, Carbs: 44.8g, Fats: 1.5g

66.   Watercress Basil Juice

Ingredients:

1 cup of watercress, torn

1 cup of basil, torn

5 plum tomatoes, halved

1 large green bell pepper

1 large cucumber

A handful of spinach

Preparation:

Combine watercress, basil, and spinach in a colander. Wash thoroughly under cold running water. Drain and torn with hands. Set aside.

Wash the plum tomatoes and place them in a bowl. Cut in half and reserve the juice while cutting. Set aside.

Wash the green bell pepper and cut in half. Remove the seeds and chop into small pieces. Set aside.

Wash the cucumber and cut into thick slices. Set aside.

Now, process watercress, basil, plum tomatoes, spinach, green bell pepper, and cucumber in a juicer. Transfer to serving glasses and stir in the salt and water.

Add some ice and serve.

Nutritional information per serving: Kcal: 112, Protein: 8.5g, Carbs: 32.7g, Fats: 1.5g

67.   Orange Pumpkin Juice

Ingredients:

1 large orange, peeled

¼ tsp of pumpkin pie spice

2 large carrots

1 small sweet potato, peeled

2 medium-sized green apples, cored

Preparation:

Peel the orange and divide into wedges. Cut each wedge in half and set aside.

Wash the carrots and chop into small pieces.

Combine all ingredients except pumpkin pie spice in a juicer and process until juiced.

Transfer the juice to serving glasses and add few ice cubes.

Sprinkle with some pumpkin pie spice and serve.

Nutritional information per serving: Kcal: 147, Protein: 2.1g, Carbs: 35.4g, Fats: 0.1g

ADDITIONAL TITLES FROM THIS AUTHOR

70 Effective Meal Recipes to Prevent and Solve Being Overweight: Burn Fat Fast by Using Proper Dieting and Smart Nutrition

By

Joe Correa CSN

48 Acne Solving Meal Recipes: The Fast and Natural Path to Fixing Your Acne Problems in Less Than 10 Days!

By

Joe Correa CSN

41 Alzheimer's Preventing Meal Recipes: Reduce or Eliminate Your Alzheimer's Condition in 30 Days or Less!

By

Joe Correa CSN

70 Effective Breast Cancer Meal Recipes: Prevent and Fight Breast Cancer with Smart Nutrition and Powerful Foods

By

Joe Correa CSN